Making Kitchen Medicines, A Pr

By Ellen Evert Hopman

MW00761896

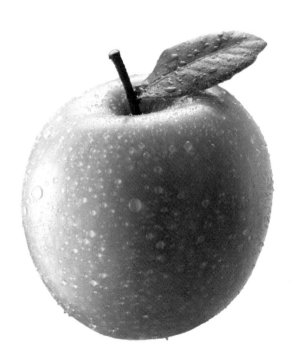

Published by Dreamz-Work Productions, LLC
4306 Independence Street
Rockville, MD 20853
USA
www.dreamz-work.com

*The recommendations found in this book have not been evaluated by the Food and Drug Administration. They are not intended to diagnose, treat, cure or prevent any disease.

ISBN 978-0-9826533-0-2
First edition: September 2009
Printed in the United States of America

The wise healer should never be at a loss when it comes to helping themselves, their friends and family, or even a pet. Sometimes the simplest remedy will do wonders - for example, taking a hot bath will often ease the symptoms of a cold, especially if a little salt (about a cup) is added to the water.

In the past all people were taught basic herbal remedies so they could doctor themselves and their friends. By using natural remedies you will be helping to preserve an ancient art.

In this book you will find an assortment of natural remedies using easily available ingredients from the kitchen shelf. After you have mastered the use of these "home remedies" you may wish to progress to further study using medicinal plants from nature or from a local health food store (suggestions for further reading are given at the end of this booklet).

IN THE EVENT OF A MEDICAL CONDITION PLEASE CONSULT A HEALTH PROFESSIONAL BEFORE USING HOME REMEDIES.

Some basic guidelines for kitchen medicines are:

Never cook with aluminum utensils, the aluminum flakes off and can lead to health problems. Use cast iron, steel, copper or ceramic cookware only.

Be sure you simmer ingredients in a pot with a tight lid so the volatile oils won't evaporate into the air. (Do not boil the herbs or they will lose their virtue).

Herbal teas can be kept in the refrigerator for up to a week in a glass jar with a tight lid. They can also be frozen into ice cubes and stored in a bag in the freezer for later use.

Whenever possible use organic ingredients so you avoid pesticides. Fruits and vegetables must be cleaned with hot soapy water and rinsed thoroughly to remove pesticide residues (which are often oil based to make them stick to the skins of fruits and vegetables).

Dried herbs and seeds should come from commercial organic growers. It is irresponsible to purchase wild-crafted organic herbs and spices, as in many cases these are becoming endangered species in their natural habitats.

Flowers and leaves are steeped in freshly boiled water that has been removed from the stove. Roots, barks, and berries are simmered (never boiled).

Honey is not suitable for babies as it may harbor bacteria.

If any herbal preparation does not agree with you or makes you feel bad then DON'T USE IT. "An ounce of caution is worth a pound of cure".

Sleep, exercise, and healthy foods are the true keys to a long, happy life.

1. ALLSPICE

This spice comes from the unripe fruits of an evergreen tree (Eugenia pimenta - commonly known as Pimentos) that grows in South America and the West Indies. It tastes and smells a bit like cloves and is used to season meats, curries and pies. You can make a remedy for upset stomach and gas by simmering 1/2 to 3/4 teaspoon of the spice in a cup of hot water for ten minutes. Be sure you use a non-aluminum pot with a tight lid.

When the tea has cooled strain it through a coffee filter and take in a tablespoon dose. Dilute it with water if it is too strong for your taste.

If you know someone with arthritis or rheumatism they might feel better if they add three or four cups of strong allspice tea to their bath water - it is warming and it eases pain. You can also soak a washcloth in the hot tea and apply it as a compress to an arthritic joint.

2. ALMOND

Almonds and dates were once the only foods eaten by camel drivers when they crossed the deserts. Almonds make a healthy survival food and may even help prevent cancer. Almonds are high in protein, Vitamin A, E, and B1, calcium, phosphorus, magnesium, folic acid and potassium.

Almond milk can be made by soaking the almonds overnight in water and then blending and straining out the milk. Add the almond milk to barley gruel or barley water (see Barley section below) as a food for invalids with kidney, bladder and gall bladder conditions.

Almond milk can be used on cereal for those with milk intolerance.

Sift together 4 oz. Almond meal, 4 oz. Rice flour and ½ oz. Orris Root powder to make a soothing skin powder.

3. ALOE

Aloe can grow in the garden in warm climates and indoors in a sunny spot in colder areas. This is a plant that you will want to have somewhere near the kitchen.

Whenever someone gets a burn, both from cooking or from the sun, split open one of the fleshy leaves and apply the moist, inner gel to the burn. Aloe is cooling and soothing and loaded with skin healing vitamins.

4. ANISE SEEDS

Anise is a spice that was used by the ancient Egyptians, Greeks and Romans. Anise seeds are used to flavor pies, cookies and stews. The tea is a great remedy for colic, gas and indigestion. It can also be taken with honey for a cough.

Steep two teaspoonfuls in a pint of freshly boiled water in a tightly covered non-aluminum pot, for ten minutes. Strain and take a tablespoonful as needed. Sweeten with honey if desired.

5. APPLE

"An apple a day keeps the doctor away" is a wise saying. In a University of Michigan study it was determined that students who ate two apples a day had fewer headaches and emotional upsets as well as clearer skin. Eating raw apples increases saliva, stimulates the gums and cleans the teeth - leading to better dental health.

Eating raw, peeled apples will help cure diarrhea. Eating apples with the skin on will ease constipation (cooked or raw). For constipation it is wise to drink plenty of extra water too.

If someone has been taking antibiotics it is a good idea to follow up afterwards with apple cider, garlic, plain yogurt, sauer kraut, or miso soup, to re-grow the correct bacteria in the intestines. Antibiotics kill friendly bacteria as well as unfriendly bacteria in the body and balance needs to be restored.

In Norse mythology it is said that when the Gods feel they are beginning to grow old they eat a diet of apples, to restore their strength and youth.

The best apples to eat are the organic green 'Granny Smith' variety. These have the least impact on blood sugar.

Do not eat the seeds as they contain cyanide, which is a poison.

6. ARTICHOKE

Artichokes can be boiled and eaten as a vegetable, just cut off the stem and sit the base of the green flower head in a pot with about 1/2 cup water - or in a steamer. But did you know that the water left over from cooking could be used medicinally?

A strong tea of the leaves is a diuretic (makes you pee) and very useful for liver problems such as jaundice. You can use a mixture of 1/2 artichoke leaves and 1/2 asparagus. Use about one pint of water for every 2 tablespoons full of vegetable matter. Simmer for 5 minutes, cool and strain and take 1/2 cup every 4 hours. Be sure to drink the tea 2 hours before a meal. (Caution: diabetics should avoid this remedy).

7. ASPARAGUS

Asparagus spears should be simmered quickly, or steamed, for no more than 5 minutes. In this way they retain their vitamins; A and C, and minerals; calcium, phosphorus, sodium, chlorine, sulfur and potassium.

Asparagus is a diuretic (makes you pee) and helpful for kidney problems. It also helps flush uric acid out of the system. Uric acid accumulates when you eat too much meat. Too much of it in the body can lead to gout and rheumatism.

(Caution: diabetics should take care with this and all diuretics)

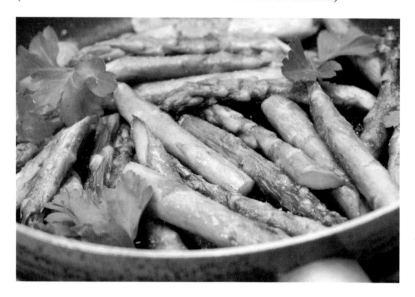

8. BANANA

Bananas are fruits of the tropical rainforests; the Earth's oldest living ecosystems. Many of the fruits and vegetables we eat originated there. Rainforests now cover only 2 % of the Earth's surface yet they are the home to over half the animal and plant species on our planet.

Rainforest fruits and vegetables include; avocados, bananas, black pepper, brazil nuts, cayenne pepper, cashews, cocoa, cinnamon, cloves, coconut, coffee, cola, corn, eggplant, figs, ginger, jalapeno peppers, lemons, oranges, papaya, paprika, peanuts, pineapple, rice, winter squash, sweet pepper, sugar, tomato, turmeric, vanilla, and yams (for more on this see Caulfield, Catherine, In The Rainforest). The medicines of the future will come from rainforests.

Bananas are best eaten when they show a few brown spots. They are loaded with vitamins; A, B, G, and riboflavin, and minerals; potassium, magnesium, sodium and chlorine. The minerals found in bananas replace the ones lost in diarrhea. Children with diarrhea will be able to keep up their weight and energy levels if they eat bananas.

In Sri Lanka a cup of the sap of the banana tree is given to a person who has been bitten by a venomous snake.

9. BARLEY

Barley is a soothing, cooling, mucilaginous (slippery) grain that is helpful in bowel diseases, throat and stomach problems, and fevers.

It can be eaten as a vegetable or if a person is very sick, given as a drink. To make barley tea first wash the barley carefully in cold water. Then boil 2 ounces of barley in one cup water for 3 minutes and strain out the liquid. Add 4 pints of fresh water and continue to boil until 1/2 of the liquid remains. Cool and strain.

Be sure you use whole grain barley because it will have all the B vitamins, calcium, magnesium, phosphorus, potassium and sodium.

10. BASIL

Basil is used in Italian recipes such as spaghetti sauce. It can be added to egg and cheese dishes and to fresh salads. It is easily grown in the garden.

Basil tea is delicious when combined with a little fresh or dried peppermintor catnip leaf and honey.

Basil tea is said to help rheumatism. It also soothes stomach upset and constipation. It has even been used to relieve whooping cough.

For headaches dip a cloth into a strong batch of basil tea and apply it to the forehead as a compress. [It works even better if you add 2 tablespoons of Witch Hazel extract. Witch Hazel is a small tree that blooms in the fall with crinkly yellow flowers].

Use one teaspoon of basil for each cup of water. Bring the water to a boil, remove from the stove, and add the basil. Allow the basil to steep for 10 minutes in a non-aluminum pot with a tight lid.

11. BEANS

The pods of beans (kidney beans, pinto beans, navy beans, green beans, snap beans, wax beans, etc.) have a lot of silica which means they help strengthen internal organs.

The pods are slightly diuretic and they also help lower blood sugar levels. They are helpful in very mild cases of diabetes. For this purpose you have to eat 9 - 16 pounds of the pods a week, cooked like a vegetable. The pods should be picked before the beans are fully ripe and are best used fresh.

The dried pods can be taken as a tea for rheumatism, kidney and bladder ailments and excess uric acid. The tea is also useful for acne. Put three handfuls of the dried, cut up pods in 1 quart of water and simmer for 3 hours in a non-aluminum pot with a tight lid.

12. BEETS

Did you know that you could eat beets raw? Grated, raw, fresh beets and carrots can be served with a little lemon juice, olive oil and sea salt. The green leaves can be steamed or lightly sautéed. Beets are loaded with vitamins such as A, B, C, and G along with plenty of blood building minerals. Beets should be taken if anemia is a problem or after an operation where a person has lost a lot of blood.

If you have a juicer you can peel the beets and put them through the machine. (Adding some carrots makes the flavor sweeter). If you don't have a juicer, peel the beets and mince them and then place them in a glass jar. Sprinkle lightly with a little sea salt and just barely cover the beets with fresh, cold water. Allow to sit for six hours and then strain out the juice. You can add more cold water to the drink if desired and adjust for taste.

13. BLACKBERRY

Blackberry is a great cure for diarrhea. You can gather the fresh leaves and pour boiling hot water over them using one pint of water per ounce of leaf. Allow the tea to get cold and strain. Take a quarter cup four times a day, in-between meals. You can also use the tea as a sore throat gargle (add a little honey if desired).

You can also dig up the roots and wash them carefully in warm soapy water. Then chop them into small pieces and simmer in a non-aluminum pot with a tight lid for 20 minutes using 2 tablespoonfuls of roots per cup of water. Strain and drink a quarter cup four times a day, not with meals. The root tea can also be used as a gargle for a sore throat.

The fresh fruits of the blackberry have similar qualities. For diarrhea you can simmer the berries in water (add just enough water to barely cover the berries) for ten minutes, mash lightly, strain out the juice and add a little brown sugar. Allow to cool and store in the refrigerator. (This remedy is especially good for babies and very small children).

A poultice of blackberry leaves can be placed on a burn or a scald. Cook the leaves slightly in just enough water to make them wilt. Cool and apply to the burn. Leave them on for about an hour and then discard. Hint: to keep a poultice in place try wrapping clear plastic wrap around it and fasten with a bit of masking tape.

14. BLUEBERRY

Blueberry syrup is another good remedy for diarrhea. Add enough water to barely cover the berries and simmer them for ten minutes in a non-aluminum pot with a tight lid. Mash lightly, strain out the juice and add a little brown sugar if needed.

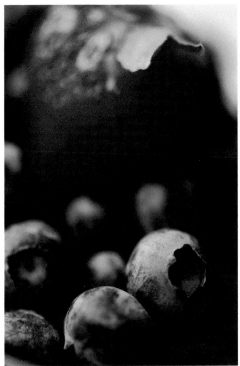

Taken over time blueberry leaf tea is said to be good for diabetics. The leaves contain myrtillin, which helps reduce blood sugar. Steep one teaspoonful of cut, dried leaves in a cup of freshly boiled water and drink up to four cups a day, not with meals.

Blueberry leaf tea can help the kidneys when a little parsley or strawberry leaf is added. The tea also strengthens the blood by adding calcium, iron, phosphorus and manganese.

15. BREAD (and other poultices)

"Cataplasma Panis" or "bread poultice" is made by crumbling up some bread and pouring boiling water over it. Allow it to sit for five minutes and then strain off the water. Place the soggy, hot bread on a clean cloth and roll out with a rolling pin until barely flat. Apply the warm poultice to sores to help clean them out, and to inflammations.

It helps to put a thick towel or flannel cloth over the poultice to keep the heat in longer. Leave on for about one half-hour. Remove the poultice when it is cold and discard.

You can also make a poultice using breadcrumbs, hot milk and freshly sautéed, chopped onion or a little grated ginger. This one is especially useful to poultice the lungs. Another simple poultice for the lungs is freshly mashed tofu with freshly grated ginger added. Warm slightly in a pot, roll out on a thick cloth and apply to the lungs when there is congestion, fever, bronchitis, etc. Grated fresh carrots can also be cooked until soft, rolled out on a clean cloth, and used to poultice the lungs. Add a little grated, fresh ginger before you cook the carrots.

16. BUTTER

The ancient Greeks and Romans had butter but they didn't eat it*. They used it externally as a skin remedy. A little butter is a quick remedy for a slight burn (not for a serious burn) or for dry skin.

The Hindus melt down butter and clarify it (by heating it gently until it is liquid and then using cheesecloth to strain out the white globs of fat and cholesterol) which is a much healthier way to eat it. Clarified butter keeps well in a glass jar with a tight lid in the refrigerator.

Hindus also offer this liquid, clarified butter (called ghee) to the Gods as a gift by pouring a little bit on a sacred fire.

An old Celtic custom is to put out a warm dish of mashed potatoes or oatmeal with a big lump of golden butter in the middle of it (symbolic of the sun) as a gift for the Fairies on the Solstices and Equinoxes.

*The ancients dipped their bread in olive oil.

17. CABBAGE

To make a cough syrup cut and slice a red cabbage. Place the sliced leaves in a glass jar and do not add any liquid. Place the jar in a pot of water and bring to a boil. Boil for three hours and then remove the jar from the pot. Strain out the liquid and add honey to taste. It should have the consistency of thick paste. Take a teaspoon as needed for a cough.

Cabbage is full of vitamins such as A, B, C and U also calcium, iodine, potassium, chlorine and sulfur. Cabbage is best eaten raw or as juice, not cooked. The outer leaves, which people often throw away, have the greatest concentrations of vitamins and calcium.

Fresh cabbage juice has been shown to help cure stomach ulcers because vitamin U protects the stomach from pepsin. This vitamin is also found in other fresh greens but is destroyed by cooking.

Dip a fresh leaf in very hot water and apply to an abscess (infection where pus is present) as a healing poultice.

18. CARAWAY

To make an antacid that helps upset stomachs, colic and gas in grownups, infants and children:

Take one half teaspoon each of caraway seeds, fennel seeds, peppermint leaf and spearmint leaf. Place in a cup and pour boiling hot water over the herbs. Cover the cup with a plate and steep for ten minutes. Stir well, strain and take one cup four times a day, not with meals.

Hint: if you have a mortar and pestle you can place the seeds into it and pound them. They will release more of their medicinal virtues this way.

Powdered caraway seeds made into a paste with a little water can be applied to bruises to heal them.

19. CARROT

Carrots are full of vitamin A, which is beneficial to the eyes, the lungs and the skin. They also help build the immune system, which helps prevent diseases such as cancer. Everyone should eat raw carrots and carrot juice on a regular basis.

Carrots can be simmered just enough so they can be mashed. Apply the cooked, mashed carrots to sores and ulcers as a poultice.

You can make a carrot salve by simmering grated carrots in olive oil. Grate a few carrots into a non-aluminum pot and just barely cover them with good quality cold pressed olive oil (count how many cups of olive oil you have used). Bring to a simmer (do not boil!) and simmer with a tight lid for about twenty minutes. (Olive oil is one of the best oils for internal and external use; plain olive oil can relieve itching)

Melt bee's wax on the stove in a separate pot. Be very careful because it is extremely flammable. Do not do this without adult supervision! (Bee's wax has propolis which is a natural skin healing agent).

When the simmering is complete remove the pot of carrots from the stove and add three tablespoons of hot, melted beeswax for every cup of oil used. Stir and then strain into very clean glass jars. Close with a tight lid and store in the refrigerator.

Apply the carrot salve to sores, burns and ulcers, but not to deep wounds where there is broken skin.

Hint: In spring and summer you can gather comfrey leaf, pine needles, plantain leaves, young oak leaves, young maple leaves, or young elder leaves and add them to the carrot salve. (see directions for salve making below)

20. CAYENNE

Cayenne pepper is a very hot red powder that is often found on the kitchen shelf. It is used to make chili and curries and is added to Mexican dishes. If someone accidentally cuts himself or herself in the kitchen you can pour powdered cayenne directly on the wound to make it stop bleeding. Men will find it useful for shaving cuts as well.

In the winter you can sprinkle a little cayenne pepper into your shoes or ice skates to help keep your feet toasty warm.

You can make a liniment (a rub for sore or arthritic muscles and joints) by mixing one part powdered red pepper, 3 parts powdered mustard, and three parts liquid soap in 10 parts of alcohol. Put the mixture into a bottle with a tight cap, shake vigorously and apply to the affected area.

Ants HATE red pepper. Make a mixture of equal parts Cayenne pepper and powdered Borax. Spread it in a line along doorways, windows, or wherever the ants come into the house.

DON'T GET CAYENNE PEPPER INTO YOUR EYES! It won't hurt your eyes but it will sting like crazy. If you do get it into your eyes flush them immediately with a strong continuous spray of cold water. It also might make some people sneeze.

21. CELERY

Celery has magnesium and iron, which strengthen blood cells. It also has elements of the B complex, vitamins that help the nerves.

If someone you know is very nervous and having trouble sleeping, frequent headaches or other signs of tension you might be able to help them with a little fresh celery and lettuce juice several times a day.

Carefully clean a few celery stalks and lettuces leaves and put them through the juicer or blend them with a little water and strain out the liquid. Take about a wineglassful between meals. Celery juice mixes nicely with carrot juice or apple cider.

22. CHERRY

Cherries should be eaten raw, not canned. Eating half a pound of fresh cherries daily has been shown to help gout and arthritis. As with all pigmented (colored) foods, cherries help build the immune system. Cherries and all other berries should be eaten freely in summer when they are easily available.

Cherries can be made into a cough and cold remedy that also helps lower fever. Take whole, very ripe, dark red cherries and stew them in a little water until soft. Squeeze out the pulp using cheesecloth and add equal parts honey. One teaspoon an hour is taken as needed.

Even the stems have value. Place a large handful of stems in a non-aluminum pot with two cups of water and simmer for twenty minutes. Strain, add honey and take a tablespoonful an hour as needed for asthma or bronchial coughs.

23. CHIVES

Chives are a type of onion grass that is grown in the garden and used as a spice. They can be harvested and cut up with scissors and stored in a plastic baggie in the freezer. One clump of chives can be harvested several times over the summer. They have vitamins C, A, B, and G and blood building minerals such as sulfur and iron.

Chive tea makes a remedy for colds and flu - steep two teaspoons of the chopped or cut up leaves in a cup of very hot water for about ten minutes. (Freeze cut chives for use in winter)

Chives, onions and garlic all help croup, asthma and coughs. Use them alone or in combination to make a cough syrup by chopping and sautéing them until soft and then adding honey. Strain and use as needed.

Chives, like garlic, have sulfur, which is bactericidal (kills germs). Add a sprinkling of chopped chives to soups and salads, potato and egg dishes to help prevent disease.

In Romania the Gypsies hang a bunch of chives, with their bulbs still attached, in the sick room to protect against evil eye and other catastrophes.

24. CINNAMON

Cinnamon is the fragrant inner bark of a tree that grows in Sri Lanka and other tropical areas.

Cinnamon water helps with chronic indigestion and gas. Put one quarter teaspoon of the ground bark into a cup of freshly boiled water, stir, cover, and allow to steep for fifteen minutes, strain and drink.

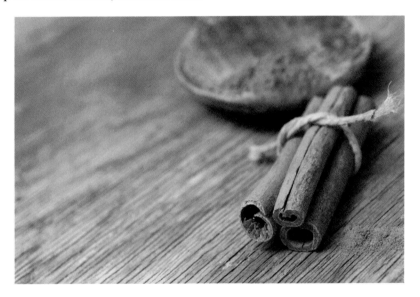

Cinnamon tea is very helpful for diarrhea and to stop vomiting. Simmer a quarter teaspoon of the ground bark or a small piece (about 1/4 inch) of cinnamon stick in a cup of water for ten minutes, strain and drink.

25. CLOVE

Cloves are actually the dried flower buds of a plant that grows in tropical areas. Cloves aid digestion and they are often stuck into foods like cooked apples and peaches and ham.

For gas and indigestion you can place three whole clove buds in a cup and pour freshly boiled water over them, steeping for ten minutes and then sipping the tea.

If you like black tea you can flavor it with a few buds of clove and a small stick of cinnamon in the pot. Another thing to add is a little cut up ORGANIC orange peel. (Never use the peels of conventionally grown oranges, lemons, limes, etc., as they will contain too much pesticide!)

Cloves can be used as aromatherapy - place a few cloves in a vaporizer or in a dish of hot water placed on a radiator. They will fragrance the room.

26. CORIANDER

The ancient Egyptians and Greeks used coriander seeds as food and medicine. The ancient Romans brought them to Britain. The Chinese say it is an herb that confers immortality.

You can make coriander water to help with gas. Steep 2 teaspoonfuls in a cup of freshly boiled water for ten minutes. Take 1/4 cup four times a day.

27. CORN SILK

Did you know that the silky hairs found at the tip of a fresh ear of corn are actually good to eat? (Be sure to only use organic corn as standard commercial corn has been sprayed with pesticides).

Fresh corn silk can be eaten in salads and is very strengthening to the bladder and kidneys.

28. CRANBERRIES

Cranberries grow in bogs in New England. Being highly pigmented (colored) they help build the immune system. Pigmented foods like red apples, red grapes, berries, red peppers, and tomatoes have the most bio-flavinoids.

In olden days sailors, who were often out at sea for months with no access to fresh fruits and vegetables, ate cranberries raw to prevent "scurvy", a disease of vitamin C deficiency. (They also ate limes for the same reason, which is why sailors were sometimes called "limeys").

Cranberry juice can help heal a bladder infection. Another way to help heal a bladder infection is to grind the berries in a food processor and add a little honey then mix the berries with plain yogurt and eat some every day. Cranberries prevent adherence of bacteria to the membrane surface of the urethra and bladder. Adding vitamin C to the diet along with the cranberries will acidify the urine even more. Cranberry juice also helps pimples, bad skin, and high blood pressure.

A poultice of mashed cranberries can be applied to boils, piles, and other skin eruptions and infections. Mash the fresh berries (or frozen ones that have been thawed out) and spread them on a clean cloth and apply. Leave the poultice on for an hour and then discard. Repeat daily until the skin is healed.

29. CUCUMBER

For severe cases of acne try a cucumber and oatmeal diet. Take nothing but cooked oatmeal with chopped up cucumbers added (skin and all) for up to three weeks. (Cook the chopped cucumbers with the oatmeal).

Cucumbers can help promote hair and nail growth due to their high silica and sulfur content. Mix cucumber juice with the juice of carrots, lettuce and spinach for this purpose. This juice will also help clear the skin.

Cucumber and carrot juices mixed together are helpful to flush excess uric acid from the system. Uric acid accumulates due to eating too much meat and it can lead to gout and rheumatic conditions.

Cucumbers have a lot of potassium, which helps regulate blood pressure, whether it is too high or too low. Cucumber salad helps chronic constipation.

Cucumber salve is great for chapped skin, dry skin and minor skin irritations;

Take 3 1/2 ounces of fresh cucumber juice and slowly beat it with a whisk into a pot with 2 ounces of melted suet. (Suet is animal fat that you can buy in the supermarket). Set the pot aside in a cold water bath and allow the ointment to solidify.

When you have an ointment like consistency pour off any coagulum on the top and put the salve into a very clean glass jar. Pour a little rose water over the salve to keep it moist and to prevent access to air. Place a tight lid on the jar and store in the refrigerator.

You can also rub the juice of cucumbers directly onto the skin to help heal burns, inflammations, bed sores and other skin irritations.

30. CUMIN

Cumin is a spice that aids digestion and helps expel gas.

Cumin is very healthy for pigeons and cures a pigeon disease known as "scabby back and breast". Take equal parts caraway, cumin, dill and fennel seeds mixed with just enough flour and a little water so you can make little cakes. Bake the cakes in the oven until firm and feed them to the birds.

Other recipes for the same condition recommend adding a little sea salt, powdered clay and asafetida to the mixture.

31. CURRANTS

Black currants can be used several different ways for healing. The juice of the berries can be simmered with sugar and used for sore throats. Simmer the berries until soft (or use the fresh juice). Add sugar and simmer again until the sugar melts. This liquid is helpful for children who have fever, sore throat, bronchitis, or whooping cough.

The berries and their juice will also benefit kidney problems and colic pains, bleeding gums and mouth and throat inflammations. The berry juice can be taken in tablespoon doses throughout the day, as needed. It is a good remedy to lower fevers.

Simmer two teaspoons of fresh berries (or one of dried) for ten minutes in a cup of water to make a gargle or mouthwash. Use 1/4 cup every hour. Adding a pinch of ground cinnamon will make the gargle even more effective.

Steeping the leaves can make a tea, which helps the kidneys, and benefits gout, whooping cough and rheumatism. It can be taken cold to soothe the throat. Steep two teaspoons of fresh (or one of dried) leaf per cup of water for ten minutes and take up to a cup a day.

A decoction of the young roots is very helpful in fevers. Carefully clean and chop the roots, using two teaspoons per cup of water simmer for twenty minutes in a non-aluminum pot with a tight lid. Take 1/4 cup between meals.

The tea of the roots can be given to cattle with dysenteric fever.

Red currant berries, which are high in vitamin C, also help lower fevers.

Prepare the berry tea as above.

32. DATES

When camel caravans crossed the deserts in ancient times they often took only dates, almonds (which provide protein) and water with them for food. These things kept them going for months.

Dates have calcium, which builds bone and muscle and strengthens the teeth and the nerves. They also have vitamins A, B, D, G and minerals such as iron, chlorine, copper, magnesium, phosphorus, potassium, sulfur and sodium.

Dates are laxative. You can boil six dates in a pint of water and drink the liquid warm, or eat six of them and follow with a glass of warm water to help constipation. Take this drink twice a day. The date water also helps piles, poor circulation, and nervousness.

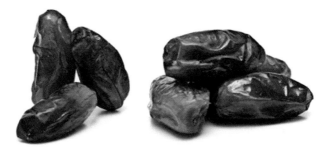

33. DILL

Dill weed (the green leaves) and seeds are added to pickles, egg dishes, salmon, beans, cauliflower, cabbage and peas.

The seeds are the most potent part, medicinally. Take equal portions of dill seeds, anise seeds and fennel seeds and using one half teaspoon of seeds per cup of freshly boiled water allow to steep for twenty minutes. This tea will help nausea, upset stomach, and gas.

For babies and young children who have colic: steep 1/2 teaspoonful of the seeds in a cup of very hot water, for six minutes. Strain and put in the baby's bottle or give with a spoon. A baby can take two to four ounces of this tea.

For gas try a mixture of 1/4 teaspoon each anise, dill, fennel seed and catnip leaf, per cup of water. Steep in freshly boiled water for twenty minutes and take a cupful four times a day, not with meals. Eat very little food throughout the day. (Catnip may drive your cats crazy but it is very relaxing for humans!)

34. EGGS

Save your eggshells! Store them until dry and them pound them to a powder using your mortar and pestle. Apply the powder to the earth around houseplants, garden plants and rose bushes. Or you can bury them whole in the soil around your plants. Eggshells have minerals that will keep your garden healthy and strong.

Eggs make a natural hair conditioner. Wash your hair with shampoo and rinse. Then apply a well-beaten raw egg to the hair and scalp, allowing it to remain on the hair for five minutes. Rinse twice to make sure all the egg is out. For dry and damaged hair you can repeat the process (but only shampoo once).

Burn remedy: beat one egg yolk with 2 ounces of flax seed oil or one egg white with 3 ounces of the oil. Apply to kitchen burns, sunburn, minor scalds, etc.

35. FENNEL

According to Pliny, an ancient Roman herbalist and naturalist, snakes rub themselves against fennel stalks as they rub off their old skins. They also sharpen their eyesight with the juice by rubbing against the plant.

According to tradition, hanging a bunch of fennel over the door on Midsummer Eve will repel evil (the herb Saint Johnswort will do the same thing, you can hang them together or alone).

When added to oily fish (salmon and mackerel) and other meat dishes during cooking, fennel helps digestion. The seeds, roots and leaves were used in ancient times as a weight loss aid, in soups and drinks.

Fennel tea, made by steeping a teaspoon of bruised seeds in a pint of hot water for twenty minutes, helps gas, hiccups, nausea (see dill).

Add some fennel seeds to your bird's food.

36. FIG

Dried figs, dates, and other dried fruits should be eaten instead of candy. But be sure to brush your teeth afterwards because the sticky fruits will cling to your teeth, causing bacteria, and cavities to grow.

Fresh figs are slightly laxative. Do not eat too many or you might get diarrhea.

Figs can be used as a poultice for boils and abscesses. Split one open and soak for a few minutes in a bowl of hot water. Then apply the fruit directly to the inflammation.

Stewed figs can be taken for a sore throat, cough, temporary constipation and upset stomach. Simmer fresh or dried figs until very soft and liquid (for about 10 minutes), strain out the juice and drink when cool. Sip half a cupful morning and evening, not with a meal.

37. GARLIC

In ancient times when poor people had no access to doctors, garlic was one of the most important cure-alls. Added to soups it can help cure colds, fevers, and flu. Mashed, fresh garlic can be applied to a wound, covered with honey (to keep out air) and then bandaged. Garlic kills viruses and bacteria.

Please don't use dried garlic capsules or genetically engineered or de-scented garlic. Old-fashioned stinky garlic is best when it comes to fighting infections.

For a sore throat or cough try putting six cloves of freshly peeled garlic in the blender with the juice of 1/2 lemon and 1/2 cup of honey.

Take in teaspoon doses as needed.

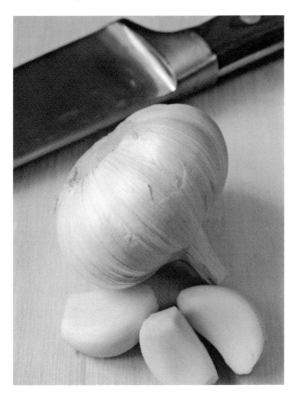

A mixture of two cups V-8 juice, juice of 1/2 fresh lemon, a few cloves of garlic, one teaspoon grated horseradish, and a pinch of cayenne pepper, blended well, will help cure a cough or cold. (Hint: the horseradish helps open blocked sinuses. Add more if you can tolerate the taste).

Garlic helps lower blood pressure by cleaning plaque from the arteries.

Crush a few cloves of garlic and apply to poison ivy. Leave it on for about 30 minutes. (Take 2 capsules of burdock root three times a day to clear poison ivy from your blood and liver)

For bronchitis, coughs and chest congestion grate some fresh garlic cloves and mix them with an equal portion of Vaseline. Place in a pan over low heat and stir until the Vaseline has melted. Do not strain, allow the mixture to cool and apply directly to the chest and back. (You can also use onion for this but garlic is even better).

Garlic should be eaten raw and cooked for all types of lung conditions but raw is always best.

For colds try chopping a peeled clove of garlic into pill sized portions and swallowing them with water into which fresh lemon juice has been squeezed. You can also "dry roast" the cloves by placing them unpeeled, in a frying pan. Do not add oil or water. Roast slowly over low heat until the garlic cloves are soft. Remove from the stove and peel. (The garlic should be like a warm paste inside the peel). Eat freely.

Garlic has vitamins C, A, B, G, sulfur, iron and calcium. It also has "Allicin" a chemical that kills germs such as staphylococci. (It can also kill some germs that penicillin can't such as bacillus paratyphoid).

Of course, garlic repels vampires and werewolves. Hang bunches around the house, windows and doors for this purpose.

38. GINGER

Ginger is a very warming spice. The part used is the root. According to the Chinese it "causes internal secretions to flow", meaning that it loosens phlegm and other internal secretions. Ginger should always be thought of in the event of a cold or the flu. Be careful not to overdo it, however. Too much ginger tea can actually irritate the lungs. Take no more than two cups of the tea a day.

Ginger tea can be made by adding 1/2 teaspoon of dried and powdered ginger to a cup of freshly boiled water with a little honey and lemon. Another way is to cut up the fresh roots and simmer them for 20 minutes in a non-aluminum pot with a tight lid using about 1/2 inch slice of ginger for every cup of water. You can save the used ginger slices and add water a second time to make another batch.

You can use ginger tea to make "ginger beer". Make a very strong tea (using more ginger per cup of water, about 1-2 inches of root) add brown sugar, lemon and honey, and fill a glass about 1/2 full with the resulting liquid. Then fill the rest of the glass with a good quality sparkling water like Evian or Perrier.

If someone has a cold or the flu try grating fresh ginger root into a pot and adding water. Simmer for 20 minutes and strain the liquid, either into a bathtub or into a footbath.

On a very cold day eating some pieces of candied ginger will actually help keep you warm.

39. GRAPES

Grapes and grape juice are very cleansing to the blood. Red grapes, being highly pigmented, have bioflavonoids that help build the immune system. They have vitamins A, B, C, sulfur, phosphorus, potassium and magnesium.

Persons with liver and kidney ailments, constipation, skin blemishes, gout and rheumatism, tumors and cancer should eat a lot of grapes, especially alone as a meal.

40. GRAPEFRUIT

Grapefruit is loaded with vitamin C, a vitamin that is not stored by the body and needs to be replenished daily. Did you know that the most vitamin C is actually in the white rind of the skin? The same is true of lemons and oranges.

You can save the skins of carefully washed organic grapefruits, lemons or oranges and cut them up. Add a teaspoon to a cup of freshly boiled water, steeping for 20 minutes. The tea will help with a cold. IMPORTANT Do not use commercially grown, non-organic fruits for this purpose because the peels will be laden with pesticides.

Try adding a little sage and mint to grapefruit rind tea, to help break up a cold.

41. HONEY

For a cough put a half-cup of honey, the juice of half a lemon, and six peeled garlic cloves into the blender. Liquefy, strain and take in teaspoon doses.

Honey makes a great wound dressing. After carefully cleaning a wound put honey over it and then bandage it. The honey absorbs water, and germs cannot live without water.

Honey contains propolis, a substance made by bees that heals burns. Honey makes a great dressing for a burn.

To make a sore throat gargle take equal parts of honey, apple cider vinegar, and freshly boiled water and stir until the honey is fully liquid. (Do not use white vinegar, as it is too harsh on the body).

Add honey to hand lotion to heal very chapped, irritated, or dry skin.

42. HORSERADISH

A mixture of two cups V-8 juice, juice of 1/2 fresh lemon, a few cloves of garlic, one teaspoon grated horseradish, and a pinch of cayenne pepper, blended well, will help cure a cough or cold. (Hint: the horseradish helps open blocked sinuses. Add more if you can tolerate the taste).

Half a teaspoon of grated horseradish, flavored with lemon juice, can be taken twice a day for sinus conditions. Horseradish has loads of vitamin C and also helps clear mucus out of the human body.

43. LEMON

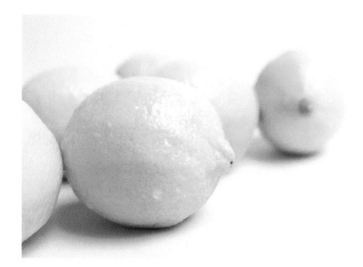

Lemons have vitamins C, B, F, P and riboflavin as well as minerals such as calcium, phosphorus, magnesium, potassium and sulfur. Lemons are very important to prevent scurvy, a disease that sailors used to get because they were out at sea for along periods with no access to fresh fruits. In England there was once a law that every ship had to carry enough lemon or lime juice so that each sailor could drink one ounce a day after being at sea for ten days.

Lemon juice mixed with honey and water helps lower a fever and adding a small bit of powdered cinnamon can help stop vomiting when someone has the flu. (See the HORSERADISH and GARLIC sections above for more ways to use lemons)

For pimples and acne try washing the face with lemon juice. Allow the juice to dry on the face; it will help dry the blemishes. Do this morning and evening. Or you can slice the lemon into very thin pieces and lay them on the skin as a face masque. Allow it to remain for 1/2 hour.

Lemon juice makes an excellent hair rinse. For dandruff try massaging the juice mixed with equal parts of water, into the scalp, allowing it to dry before shampooing. If you are lucky enough to live in a climate where lemons grow outdoors you can apply freshly squeezed lemon juice to your hair daily and keep it in while you go out in the sun. Over time it will bleach your hair.

Apply fresh lemon juice to the sting of a wasp or a bee.

For corns and bunions, bathe the foot until the skin is softened then wrap the foot in a bandage or cloth soaked with lemon juice.

Apply lemon juice to a wart frequently to make it disappear.

Lemon and grapefruit seeds can be planted in vermiculite or a mixture of sand and soil. First carefully rinse the seeds in cold water and then dry with a napkin or paper towel, then plant them. Keep the potted seeds in a sunny window, spraying them with water daily to keep them moist. When the seedlings are a few inches tall transplant them into separate pots with 2/3 sand and 1/3 soil. You will eventually have a pretty little tree.

44. LETTUCE

Lettuce leaves have vitamins C and A. The darker the lettuce the more vitamins and minerals it will contain. Lettuce, and salads in general, are a great cure for constipation. Everyone should eat at least one salad a day.

Lettuce is very calming. For insomnia try adding a few lettuce leaves to a pint of boiling water. Simmer for 20 minutes well covered, strain and drink when slightly cooled, before bed.

If someone is very nervous try putting equal parts of lettuce leaves and celery stalks into the juicer. You can also add a carrot or two for taste. They should drink this juice several times a day. (See CELERY section above).

45. MILK

A classic cure for insomnia is a cup of warm milk before bed (please use organic, raw milk without added growth hormones and antibiotics).

For severe eczema, try applying a cloth soaked in milk as a compress. It will give temporary relief of itching and pain.

If someone gets an irritating spice such as salt or pepper into their eyes first flush with water and ten apply a few drops of milk with an eyedropper into the corner of the eye.

For coughs add a teaspoon each of honey and sesame or sunflower oil to a cup of warm milk and sip slowly.

For diarrhea in children add 2 or 3 pinches of powdered cinnamon to a cup of warmed milk.

For adults double the amount of cinnamon.

Those with allergies, sneezing, or mucus congestion in the chest and sinuses should avoid milk.

Babies that are allergic to milk can eat slippery elm pudding. It has just as much calcium as cow's milk. Just mix powdered slippery elm bark with water to make the pudding. Or you can soak nuts such as almonds, hazel nuts, pumpkin seeds, etc overnight in water and blend in the morning. Strain out the nut milk.

Goat's milk is easier for humans to digest than cow's milk. It has more protein and less fat per volume.

46. MUSTARD

A mustard foot bath works wonders for colds, bronchitis and even pneumonia because it warms the body and lowers fever. For acute conditions it is best to take the footbath every two hours. If any sign of skin irritation develops stop using the footbath immediately.

A mustard footbath will also relieve pain in the sinuses, pain in the ear, and pain from ulcerated teeth (abscess). The mustard bath opens the capillaries and moves blood to the surface vessels of the body, removing tension and congestion from the sinuses, the roots of the teeth, and the ear.

To make the bath place 3-4 ounces of powdered mustard in a cloth bag and steep in a few cups of warm water for five minutes.

A mustard plaster is useful for chest colds, bronchitis and pneumonia. To make the plaster, mix one tablespoon of powdered mustard with three tablespoons of flour (rye is best). Add equal portions of apple cider vinegar and water to make a paste. Spread the paste on a cloth and apply to the chest. It will burn slightly. Remove the plaster when the burning sensation becomes uncomfortable. Thoroughly clean the skin with warm water after applying the plaster and apply a soothing lotion if necessary. In a few days the skin will return to normal.

Did you know you could use powdered mustard to remove smells from old bottles and jars? Mix up a little dry mustard and water and fill the bottle or jar. Allow the liquid to sit in the bottle or jar for several hours then rinse with very hot water.

47. OATMEAL

Oatmeal is a laxative food for those who are prone to constipation. For babies who are constipated make the oatmeal with extra water and strain out the liquid, giving it to the baby in a bottle.

Oatmeal is very digestible and should be given to those who are weak from illness and fever. It can be flavored with raisins or a little grated lemon, some sweetener and a little soymilk.

Oatmeal makes a good poultice for bruises, ulcers, and wounds. The hulls of oats contain a bactericidal substance (kills germs). To make the poultice use the oatmeal alone or mix one part oatmeal to two parts flax seed. Add enough hot water to make a paste that can be spread thickly on a cloth. Apply to the affected area and leave it on for about an hour. (Hint - tape the edges of the cloth together so the oatmeal doesn't fall out). Please use whole oats for this process, not the powdered, "instant" variety. (see "Cucumber" section above for more on oatmeal and skin healing)

48. OLIVE OIL

Olive oil is probably the healthiest oil for internal use; it benefits the heart by keeping cholesterol down. Use it in cooking and as a substitute for butter (In many countries people dip their bread in olive oil. You can also add a little chopped parsley, garlic, rosemary, or cilantro to flavor the oil)

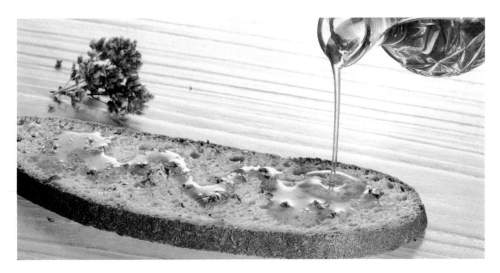

Olive oil is a wonderful skin healer. It even stops the itch of chicken pox. Apply it to stings and burns, bruises, itching, and sprains. Massage it into the chest and back of those with chest complaints (for lung conditions Sunflower oil is also excellent).

For burns and inflammations try using a mixture of equal parts olive oil and lime juice, massaging it into the skin.

Olive oil can be massaged into a joint where there is bursitis. Do this daily until full movement is restored.

Olive oil is used in salves and ointments (see carrot section above and salve making instructions below).

49. ONION

Onions are antiseptic and loaded with Vitamin C. For coughs, hoarseness, asthma, and colds, chop up a small, fresh onion and place in the blender with honey to make syrup. Take the syrup once every hour, in teaspoon doses.

A strong onion soup will benefit bronchitis and other chest conditions. Take it several times a day.

ONION SOUP

3 tablespoons butter
4 cups sliced onion
1/2 teaspoon honey
1 tablespoon flour
Salt
Ground pepper

Melt the butter in a large pot and add the onions, cooking very slowly over a low heat, stirring frequently. Add the honey and flour and cook for 3 minutes. Add 4 cups water and simmer gently in a non-aluminum pot with a tight lid, for 30 minutes. Add salt and pepper to taste.

A slice of raw onion can be applied to the sting of a bee or a wasp.

Onion juice can be applied to infected wounds. Freshly peeled onions can be placed in the blender and the resulting mash applied as a poultice.

Onions benefit the heart by lowering blood pressure.

When there is sickness in the house cut an onion in half and leave it in the sick room, replacing it daily. The onions used in this fashion should be burned or buried and never eaten, as they have become a magnet for germs.

50. ORANGE

As with grapefruits and lemons, oranges are loaded with vitamin C, but most of it is in the white rind just under the skin. Eating the white rind will help prevent colds and infections, and speed the healing of wounds.

Don't throw away your orange seeds! Plant them in a flowerpot and when the trees are about three inches high you can snip the leaves and add them to salads.

51. OREGANO

You probably think of oregano as a spice for spaghetti sauce or salads. But did you know it makes a wonderful tea? You can gather the fresh herb in the summer and put it into a plastic zip-lock bag and store it in the freezer for use all winter. It tastes best when a little peppermint leaf is added to the brew.

Oregano is great for indigestion, nausea and colic. It also helps relieve gas, lowers a fever, and is soothing to the nerves. Peppermint helps with flatulence and upset digestion and is also cooling for a fever, so they are an ideal combination.

Oregano has pain-relieving and germicidal properties due to the camphor found in its volatile oils.

Steep half a teaspoon of oregano or of a mixture of peppermint and oregano, per cup of freshly boiled, hot water. The tea can be taken internally for the conditions mentioned above, or applied externally as a compress when someone has a headache. Dip a cloth in a strong batch of the tea and apply to the face as often as needed.

You can put fresh oregano in the blender with just enough water to liquefy and then pour the mix into a bowl. Add a little powdered slippery elm bark or buckwheat flour to make a poultice for sprains, bruises, swellings and other painful conditions. Spread it on a cloth and apply to the affected area. Keep it on for an hour and discard.

If you have dried oregano and you want to make a poultice just put the dried leaves in a bowl and pour a little boiling hot water over them. Soak the leaves in the water until soft, add a little flour or slippery elm bark to make it all hold together, and then spread the poultice material on a cloth and apply.

52. PAPAYA

The Seminole Indians of Florida used fresh papaya leaves as a wound dressing. The leaves were also used to wrap meat to tenderize it. Modern meat tenderizers that you find in the supermarket are often made from dried papaya fruit and leaf.

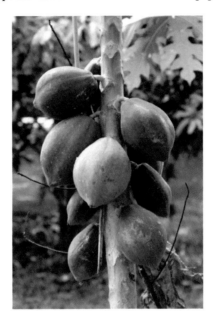

Papaya fruits are full of vitamins; A, C, E, D, K, and also calcium, phosphorus and iron. They also contain protein, citric, malic, and tartaric acids as well as sodium, potassium and phosphoric acid, plus an abundance of natural sugar but no starch. They have enzymes that help the stomach to digest other foods. If eaten regularly on an empty stomach as a fruit or liquefied and then drunk, papaya helps rebuild the entire digestive tract. Try it if you have a hard time digesting things like onions, garlic, milk or cheese.

Papaya fruit helps a body to maintain regularity, and when taken alone on an empty stomach helps remove dead tissue from the bowels and digestive tract when there is disease. It also helps the body maintain an acid-alkaline balance and removes excess mucus from the system.

53. PARSLEY

Parsley is sacred to the goddess Persephone and was used by the ancient Greeks in their funeral rites. They decorated tombs with wreaths of parsley and also used it to crown the winners in athletic contests, mostly because it kept its color for a long time. Charioteers and warriors fed it to their horses. It was such a sacred plant that it was considered disrespectful to bring it to the table!

Parsley leaves have large amounts of beta-carotene (water soluble vitamin A), vitamins C and B. They also contain trace minerals such as calcium, phosphorus, potassium, copper, iron, manganese, magnesium, sulfur, and iodine. (See WATERCRESS below)

Parsley strengthens and cleans the blood. Parsley is also cleansing to the kidneys. Steep one teaspoon of the chopped fresh or dried leaf in a cup of freshly boiled water until the water is cold. Stir, strain and drink several times a day. Parsley tea and juice have been used to help asthma, liver problems such as jaundice and coughs. For lung conditions such as bronchitis try adding parsley to fresh carrot juice.

The fresh juice can be strained and dropped into the eye to help eye inflammations such as conjunctivitis and blepharitis.

(For conjunctivitis make a strong tea of powdered goldenseal root, steep for about 10 minutes, strain through an organic coffee filter, and drop the cooled tea into the eyes three or four times a day as needed. It relieves the itch and rapidly clears the infection)

During World War I, soldiers who had kidney problems often drank parsley tea.

CAUTION: NEVER USE THE TEA IF THERE IS KIDNEY INFLAMATION PRESENT!

People with halitosis (bad breath) should make a habit of eating it as a condiment (and have a dentist check their teeth and gums).

54. PARSNIP

Parsnips are a root vegetable that looks like white carrots. They are usually boiled with a little salt, or placed in the pan when you roast a chicken. Cut up the roots along with carrots and arrange them along the sides of a roasting pan into which a chicken has been placed. Be sure to add a few inches of water.

Parsnips have chlorine, iron, magnesium, phosphorus, potassium, sulfur and silica. Parsnips help calm the nerves and strengthen the hair and nails.

Pigs, horses and cattle like to eat parsnips. They help to fatten pigs and increase milk in cows.

PARSNIP CAKES
Cook the parsnips until soft, mash with butter, add a little salt and pepper.

Take a handful of the mash and form it into a cake, then dredge in flour.

Fry in oil until slightly crisp.

PARSNIP SALAD
Take cold, cooked parsnips and slice them.

Season with salt and pepper and a Vinaigrette dressing.

55. PEACH

You can use the leaves of the Peach tree to make a tea that will help with nervous conditions, bronchitis, and chest congestion. Peach leaf tea also helps stop nausea. Be sure you get the leaves from a tree that has NOT been sprayed with insecticides.

To make the tea steep 1 tsp. of the leaf per cup of freshly boiled water and allow it to sit until cold. Take several cups a day, the first one before breakfast.

Peach leaves contain hydro cyanic acid, which makes them slightly sedative (they stop spasms such as coughing and vomiting). They are also slightly laxative, slightly diuretic (they promote bowel movements and increase urine) and expectorant.

You can gather peach leaves in early summer and dry them for later use.

Peaches have iron, which is important for the blood. They should be eaten often in summer when they are in season, alone or combined with apples, apricots, blackberries, mulberries, elderberries and blue berries.

56. PEPPER, BLACK

In ancient times black pepper was very highly prized. For example, when Attila the Hun attacked Rome he demanded 3,000 pounds of it as a ransom to liberate the city!

Black pepper can be used to make a poultice for the pain of rheumatism, sprains, nerve pain, and pleurisy.

To make the poultice put a cup and a half of apple cider vinegar into a non-aluminum pan, and bring to a boil on the stovetop. Sift in enough powdered black pepper to make a paste. Spread the paste on a piece of clean cloth large enough to cover the affected area. Leave the poultice in place for about three hours and then discard. Clean any residue off using Witch Hazel, not water (water will ruin the healing effects).

Black pepper taken internally is slightly laxative and aids digestion. It helps with nausea, gas and diarrhea.

57. POMEGRANATE

According to the prophet Mohammad eating pomegranates purges anger and jealousy out of the system.

Pomegranate juice is a "refrigerant" meaning it can actually lower body temperature. It is a great juice to drink during the heat of summer and it can also be used to lower fevers.

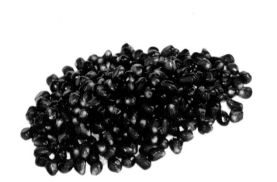 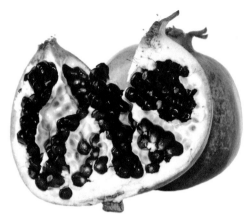

Save the seeds, dry them and powder them using your mortar and pestle. Add the powdered seeds to cough syrups; they help to remove phlegm from your system.

58. POTATO

When you eat potatoes always include the skin, as that is where the vitamins are. However, if the skin has turned green cut that section off or discard the potato, as it will then contain alkaloids, a type of poison. Did you know that potatoes are in the same family as Deadly Nightshade?

If you mix potatoes and corn together it makes a complete protein. Potatoes have citric acid, which builds the immune system and repairs tissue, and the skins have Vitamin K, which aids in blood clotting.

Grated raw potato can be applied to sprains, bruises and synovitis (a type of joint inflammation). For rheumatism, cut up some unpeeled, raw potatoes and infuse them for several hours in cold water, along with the fresh stalks and unripe berries of the potato plant. Apply the water as a cold compress to the affected part. Be sure to use only ORGANIC potato plants (to avoid pesticides).

For burns and scalds, peel a raw potato, cut it up and then and pound it into a mush with your mortar and pestle, and apply. Or just cut it into very thin slices and place those over the burn.

The inner pulp of a cooked baked potato can be mashed with a fork and then oil added, to make a remedy for frostbite.

A cooked potato poultice improves circulation, cleans the blood, helps arthritis, and clears the kidneys of toxins when placed over them. The poultice can also be placed over an infection to pull out toxins. Place it over any organ that is ailing, for example the lungs when someone has bronchitis. The poultice will help pull heat and fever out of the system.

To make a potato poultice, mash the inner pulp of cooked potatoes (do not use the skins). Get some Plantain leaves from the garden - Plantain is a very common "weed" that grows in lawns. Put the Plantain leaves in the blender with just enough water to make a "mush" out of them. You can use wheat grass or fresh Comfrey leaf if you have it, instead.

Pour the plantain mush into a bowl, add the mashed, cooked potatoes, and then gradually add flour (buckwheat is the best flour to use for poultices as people will not be allergic to it). Knead with your fingers all the while until you get a pie dough consistency.

Put the lump of poultice on a clean cloth and roll it out with a rolling pin (a little flour on the rolling pin with prevent sticking). The poultice should look like a flat pancake. Apply the poultice to the part of the body that needs it. Leave it on for an hour and then discard.

Be sure the person is warm when you do this. Apply the poultice and then cover the person with a towel (to prevent staining) and a blanket.

59. PRUNES

Prunes are actually dried plums. They are slightly laxative and should be eaten stewed by those who need help maintaining healthy bowel movements. (We all do from time to time!)

60. PUMPKIN SEEDS

Pumpkin seeds are available at your local health food store. Eating pumpkins seeds will help get worms out of your system (did you know that at any given time eighty percent of the human population has worms? We get them from walking around barefoot and from frequent contact with dogs, cats, and other animals). You will need to fast from other foods while eating the seeds. Start on an empty stomach and eat a handful of seeds every hour for three hours. Chew the seeds thoroughly.

You can also drink "pumpkin milk" at the same time, which is made by placing the seeds in the blender with cold water.

Follow with a dose of castor oil to drive out the worms. Repeat the whole process if necessary. If you have a tapeworm be sure the whole thing comes out!

Pumpkin seeds are very beneficial to the male prostate gland.

Pumpkin seed oil is soothing for burns and severely chapped skin.

61. RASPBERRY

Dried raspberry leaves make a nice tea which can be used as a sore throat gargle and as a wound wash. It also helps diarrhea. The fruits are very building to the blood and the immune system. They contain vitamin C and minerals, magnesium, calcium, phosphorus, pectin, proteins, citric acid, malic acid, sodium, chlorine, sulfur and potassium.

Eating raw raspberries (and strawberries) in the summer helps dissolve tartar on the teeth, and helps build the immune system.

To lower a fever boil a handful of the fresh berries in two cups of water for ten minutes, in a non-aluminum pot with a tight lid. Strain and cool. Half a cup of the liquid can be taken hourly.

For diarrhea, increase the amount of berries in the drink.

To benefit the heart, make syrup of raspberries by liquefying fresh raspberries in the blender and then simmering 7 parts fresh juice with 10 parts sugar. Then add one part of the syrup to two parts red wine vinegar. Take a few tablespoons of this cardiac syrup daily.

62. SAGE

The Latin name for Sage is "Salvia" meaning "to be saved", because the herb has helped so many people. Toads love this plant. It is said that the wife rules in a home where Sage prospers in the garden.

Sage is a spice used to flavor cooked turkey. It is also used in salads. Steeping two teaspoons of the leaves in a cup of freshly boiled water for half an hour makes sage tea. Take a quarter cup, four times a day, to dry up moist coughs and lung congestion. You can also use the tea as a gargle for tonsillitis, laryngitis, and sore throats.

Sage also helps with bad breath, bleeding gums, and mouth sores.

Crush the fresh leaves and apply them to insect bites and stings.

63. STRAWBERRIES

Like Raspberries, fresh strawberries help dissolve tartar on the teeth. To whiten teeth, allow the fruit to remain on them for five minutes and then brush the teeth with a mixture of water and bicarbonate of soda. The fruits are slightly laxative.

Mash the fresh fruits and apply them to the face as a masque or to treat sunburn. Leave on for half an hour and then wash the face with water, do not use soap.

(Other fruits such as apricots, banana and oatmeal with a little honey and cream mixed in also make a skin healing face masque!)

64. WATERCRESS

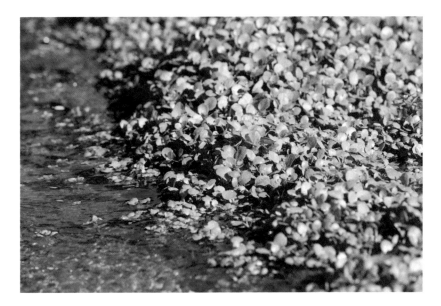

Watercress grows in streams but you can buy it in the supermarket. It is a valuable source of trace minerals and also helps clean the liver. By eating watercress and parsley often you will get just about all the minerals available from land vegetables. Only seaweeds have more blood building and tissue nourishing trace elements.

Watercress is used as a garnish and added to salads and egg dishes. Its leaves contain phosphorus, potassium, iron, manganese, fluorine, copper, sulfur, iodine and zinc.

MAKING HERBAL SALVES

Collect the green outer hulls of walnuts (they are anti-fungal and skin healing), the shiny whole nuts of horse chestnut (smash the nuts and add them to the pot/they are anti-inflammatory and stop pain) also add up to THREE of the following;
 Pine needles, plantain leaves, leaves of bee balm/Monarda, lavender flowers, calendula flowers, comfrey leaves, elecampane root, birch bark, Saint Johnswort, young oak leaves, young maple leaves, young elder leaves.

Place the herbs into a non aluminum pot with a tight lid.
Just barely cover with cold pressed olive oil. Carefully count the cups of olive oil you have used.

Bring to a simmer. Simmer for 20 minutes with the lid on (do not boil!)

In a separate pot bring bee's wax to a simmer.

When the herbs have finished simmering and the bee's wax is ALSO at a full simmer, add 3 tablespoons of hot bee's wax PER CUP

OF OIL USED.

Stir. Strain into very clean class jars.

When cool put the lid on the jars and store in a cool, dark place.

Uses; burns, sunburn, diaper rash, dry skin, chapped lips, chafing, itching, dry feet, superficial scrapes and wounds.

WARNING: DO NOT USE OIL BASED PRODUCTS ON A DEEP WOUND!

Harvesting hint: The peeled, green outer hulls of walnuts can be stored in the freezer as can the shiny brown nuts of the horse chestnut tree. Gather fresh comfrey leaves and other green herbs and flowers and freeze them in zip lock bags for later use throughout the year!

.

REFERENCES

Grieve, M., A MODERN HERBAL, Dover Publications, Inc., NY, 1971

Harris, Benjamin, F., KITCHEN MEDICINES, Natura Publications, Worcester, MA, 1961

Lust, John, THE HERB BOOK, Bantam Books, NY, 1974

Quelch, M.T., HERBAL REMEDIES, Faber and Faber Ltd., London, 1915.

BOOKS FOR FURTHER STUDY

Hopman, Ellen Evert, A Druid's Herbal of Sacred Tree Medicine, Inner Traditions Bear and Company, Rochester, VT, 2008.

Hopman, Ellen Evert, A Druid's Herbal For the Sacred Earth Year, Inner Traditions/Destiny Books, Rochester, VT, 1995

Hopman, Ellen Evert, Walking The World In Wonder – A Children's Herbal, Inner Traditions, Rochester, VT, 2000

Ellen Evert Hopman's home page: www.elleneverthopman.com

POB 219, Amherst, MA 01004 USA

INDEX

About the author

ELLEN EVERT HOPMAN

http://www.elleneverthopman.com

Ellen Evert Hopman is a Master Herbalist and lay Homeopath with an M.Ed. in Mental Health Counseling. Hopman is a founding member of The Order of the White Oak (Ord Na Darach Gile, www.whiteoakdruids.org) and its current Co-Chief. She is a professional member of the American Herbalists Guild.

Ellen Evert Hopman is the author of a growing number of books. Her first novel, Priestess of the Forest: A Druid Journey (Llewellyn, February 2008), was an exciting new project for her, combining a heart-warming fictional romance with practical Druid rites and rituals. The sequel is called The Druid Isle (Llewellyn, April 2010). Her newest book on tree medicine and tree lore is A Druid's Herbal for Sacred Tree Medicine (Inner Traditions - Bear and Company, June 2008). Other books include Being a Pagan: Druids, Wiccans, and Witches Today (Destiny Books, 2001), People of the Earth: The New Pagans Speak Out (Inner Traditions, 1995), Walking the World in Wonder - A Children's Herbal (Healing Arts Press, 2000), A Druid's Herbal for the Sacred Earth Year (Destiny Books, 1994) , and Tree Medicine -Tree Magic (Phoenix Publishing, Inc., 1992).

Hopman has presented on Druidism, herbal lore, tree lore and Celtic spirituality at conferences, festivals, and events in Northern Ireland, Ireland, Scotland, Canada, and the United States. She has participated in numerous radio and television programs including National Public Radio's "Vox Pop" and the Gary Null show in New York. She presented a weekly "herb report" for WRSI radio out of Greenfield, MA for over a year and was a featured subject in a documentary about Druids on A&E Television's "The Unexplained" (Sacred Societies, February 1999).

She has also released video tapes and DVDs on the subjects covered in her books through Sawmill River Productions. See clips at: http://vimeo.com/user2687064/videos Purchase the DVDs for $20.00 plus $4.00 from Ellen Hopman at POB 219, Amherst, MA 01004

Dreamz-Work Productions

www.dreamz-work.com

LaVergne, TN USA
04 June 2010
185042LV00001B